WHEN I LOOK INTO THE MIRROR

A Self-Esteem Builder and Diary For Women of Color

LaVon Jackson Maccanico

Copyright © 2017 by LaVon Jackson Maccanico

Published by ╬RICHER Press
An Imprint of Richer Life, LLC
2320 East Baseline Road, Suite 148-214, Phoenix, Arizona 85042
www.richerlifellc.com

Cover Design: RICHER Media USA

No part of this publication may be reproduced, stored in a retrieval system, or transmitted in any form or by any means, electronic, mechanical, photocopying, recording, scanning, or otherwise, except as permitted under Section 107 or 108 of the 1976 United States Copyright Act, without prior written permission of the publisher.

Library of Congress Control Number: 2017951238

When I Look Into The Mirror
A Self-Esteem Builder and Diary For Women of Color

LaVon Jackson Maccanico
p.   cm.

1. Diaries   2. Self-help   3. Health
ISBN 978-0-9988773-2-7
(pbk : alk. Paper)

PRINTED IN THE UNITED STATES OF AMERICA

August 2017

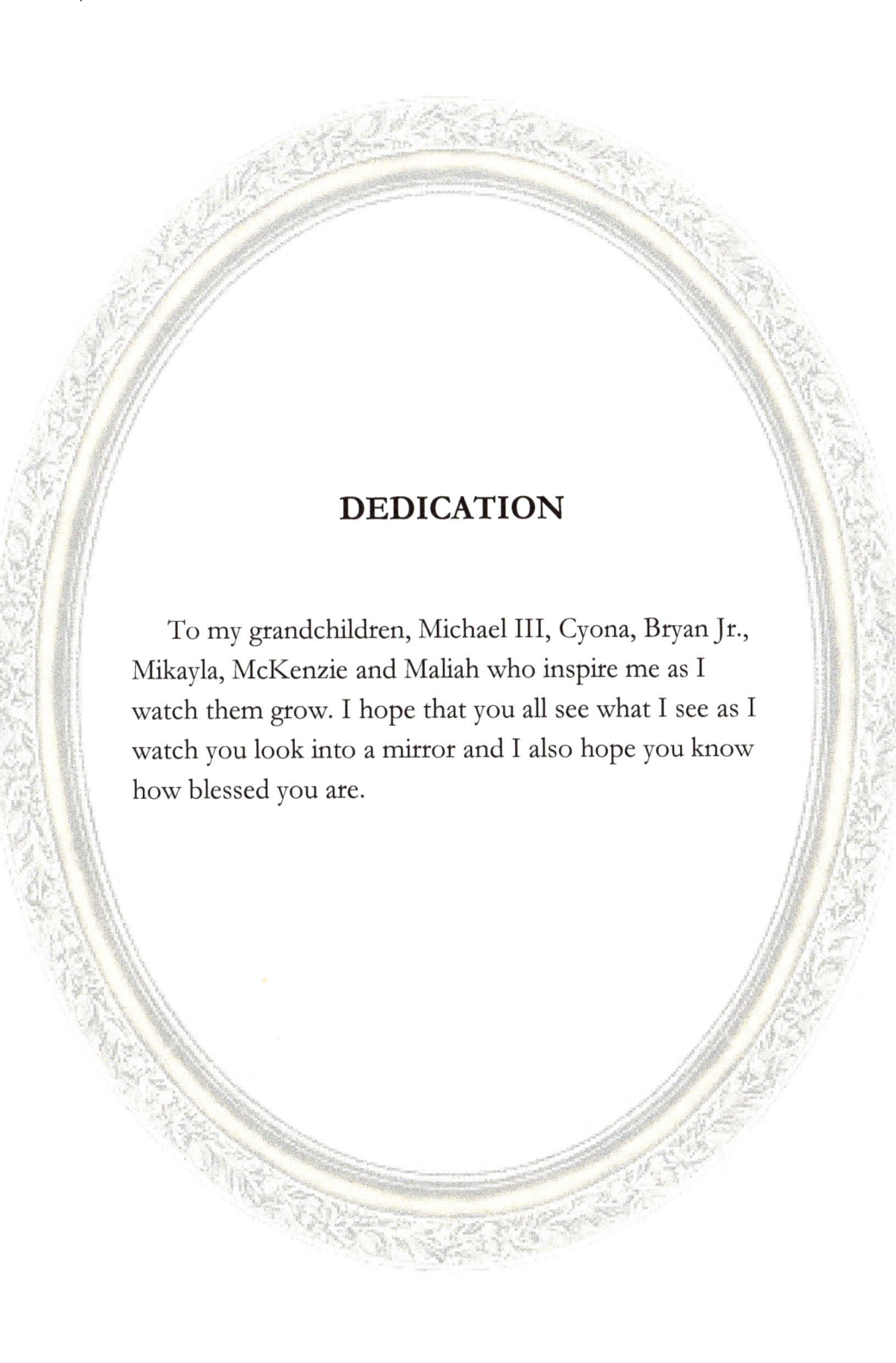

DEDICATION

To my grandchildren, Michael III, Cyona, Bryan Jr., Mikayla, McKenzie and Maliah who inspire me as I watch them grow. I hope that you all see what I see as I watch you look into a mirror and I also hope you know how blessed you are.

ACKNOWLEDGEMENTS

Thank God for the courage to publish this book. He is my Lord and Savior who guides me daily.

Moran Sr., thank you for encouraging me to follow my heart which resulted in the writing of this book.

Breanna Lienberger, thank you for your incredible insight and invaluable input on my first manuscript.

Camille Stinson, thank you for your support with the initial illustrations.

May God continue to bless all of you on this side of heaven. Thank you for your loving support.

And to my children who always listen to me and encourage me beyond my wildest dreams.

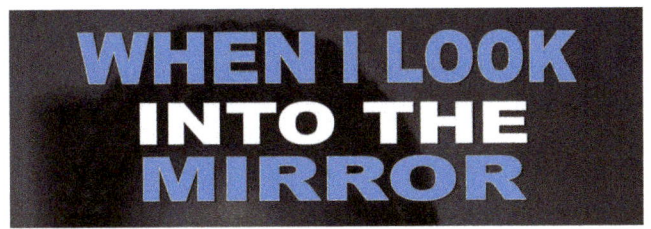

INTRODUCTION

This book is intended to help build self-esteem and increase self-awareness by utilizing the power of a routine activity we all undertake everyday...*looking into the mirror*.

Every day we all look into a mirror. However, too often we only see our own reflection and not our *inner* self.

The thoughts, messages and photographs in this book have all been carefully selected and arranged to help women of color see who they really are when they look into the mirror. As a Christian, I also personally hope that this book helps to remind you of what God sees every day.

I suggest that you take advantage of the diary pages in this book and record an honest view of what you see when you look in the mirror today...tomorrow...and the next day.

When you spend time with this book and its messages on a frequent basis, I suggest that you use the diary pages to *track the changes* that have occurred within your self, your attitude and your life as you increasingly embrace the *inner* you.

A completed diary can always be re-visited to remind yourself of how you finally arrived at seeing the *real you*. It will be a factual reminder of the *thoughts* and *fears* you carried around with you from day to day regarding your self and your earthly being.

It would be great if you would share your completed diary with your daughters, granddaughters and girlfriends to help them take advantage of your unique journey and to make them aware of the fears and doubts you too had to conquer, along the way, to find that *inner you*.

Enjoy this book and the journey as you grow, become more confident and become the best you!

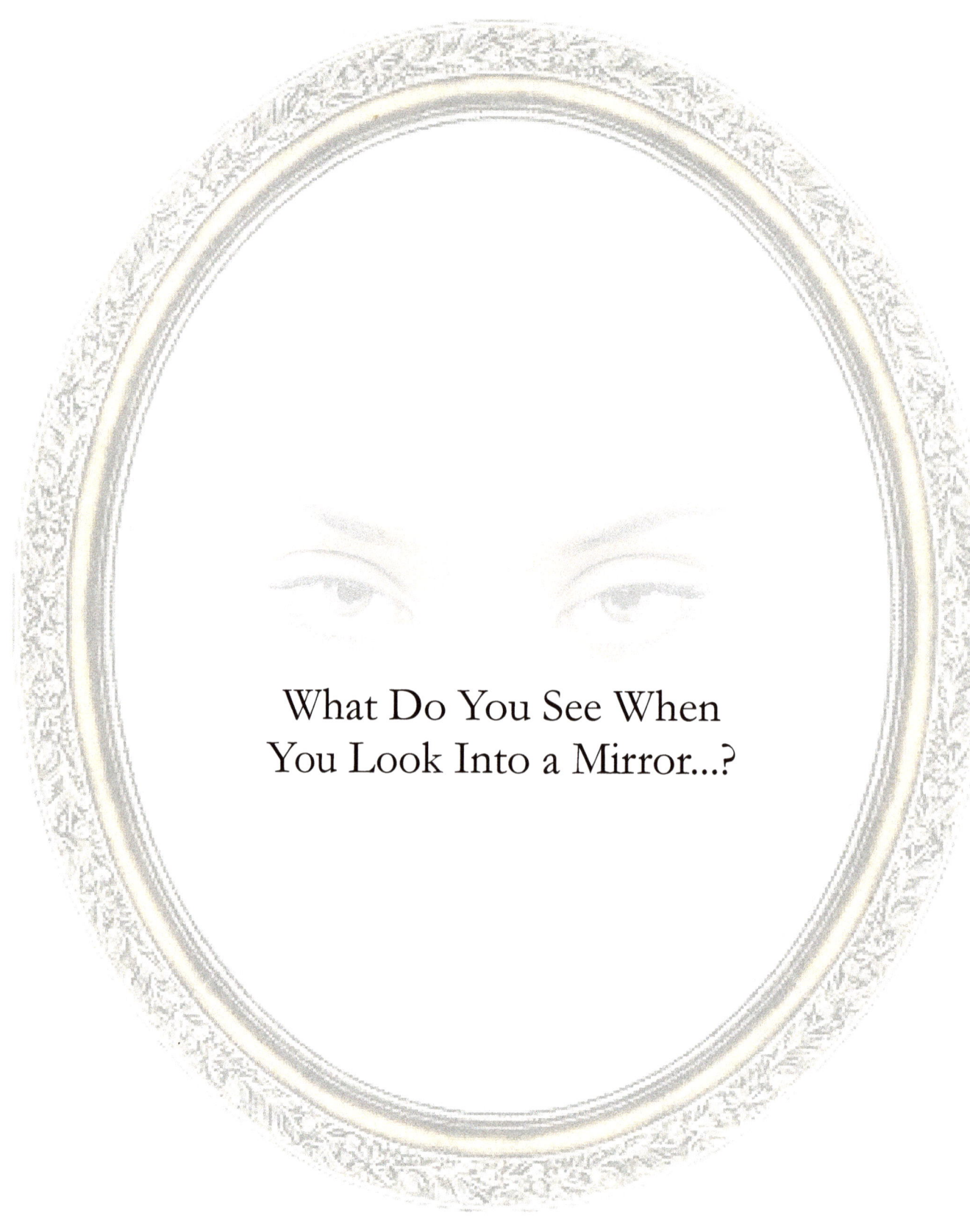

What Do You See When You Look Into a Mirror...?

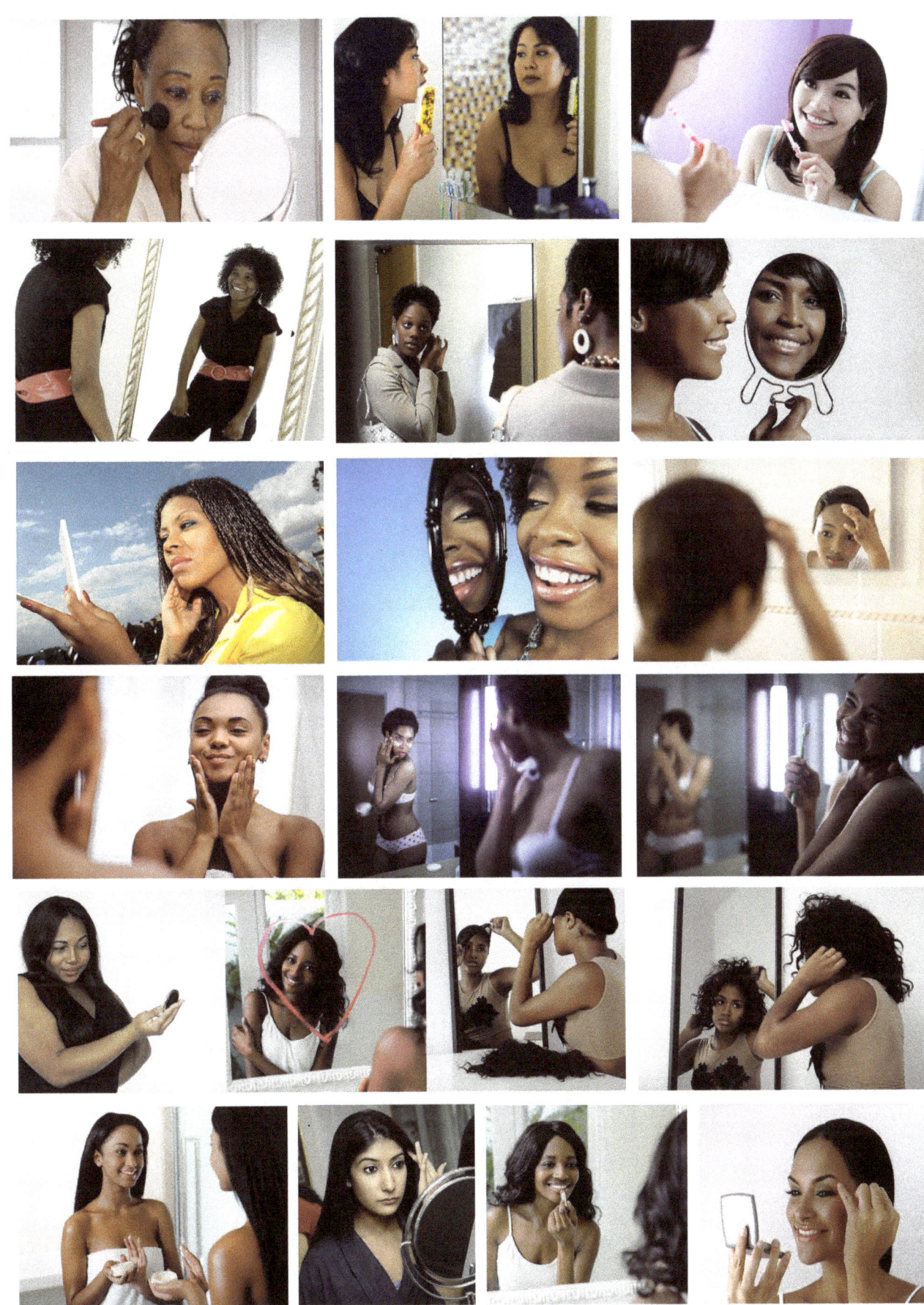

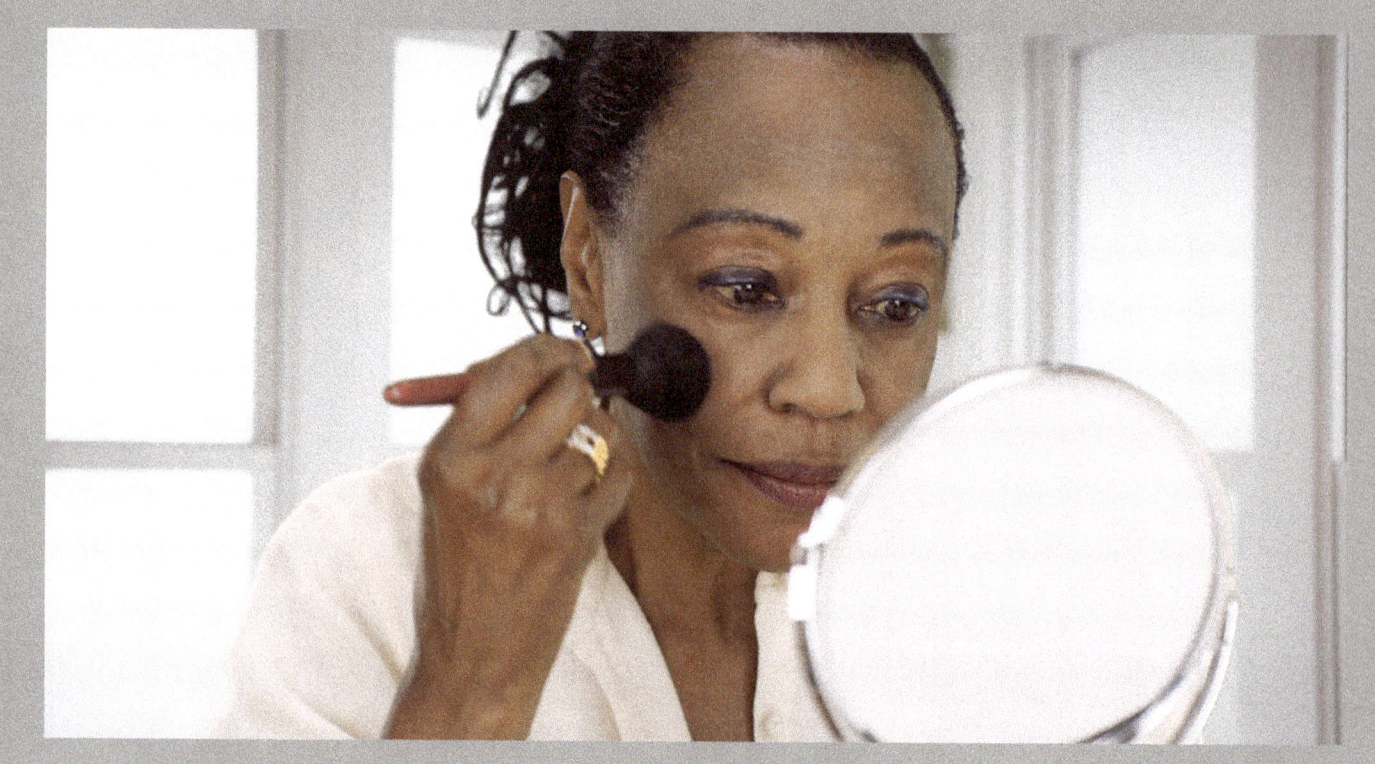

What do you see?

God himself in the flesh; that's me.

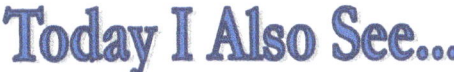

Today I Also See...

Date:

___

Date:

___

Date:

___

Date:

___

WHEN I LOOK INTO THE MIRROR

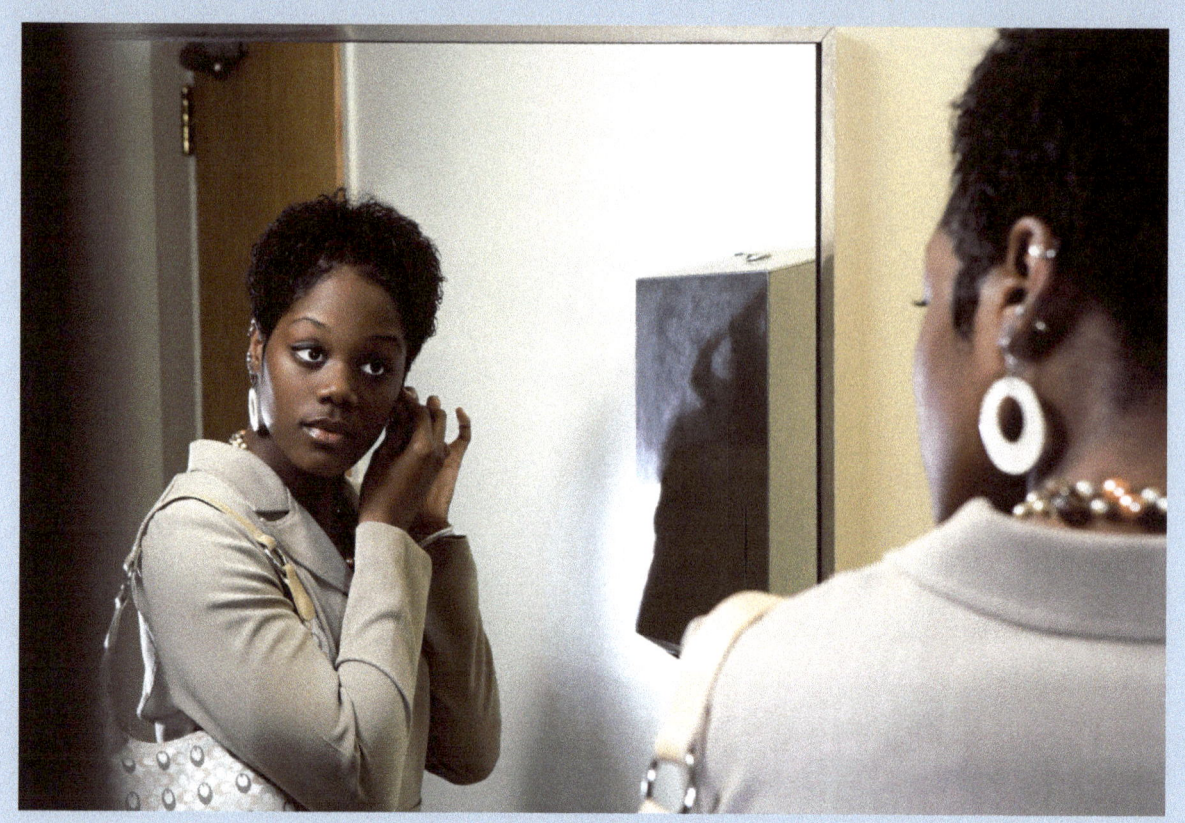

What do you see?

...A beautiful brown skinned girl thinking
God you sure look good in me.

Today I Also See...

Date:

_____
_____
_____
_____
_____
_____

Date:

_____
_____
_____
_____
_____
_____

Date:

_____
_____
_____
_____
_____
_____

Date:

_____
_____
_____
_____
_____

WHEN I LOOK INTO THE MIRROR

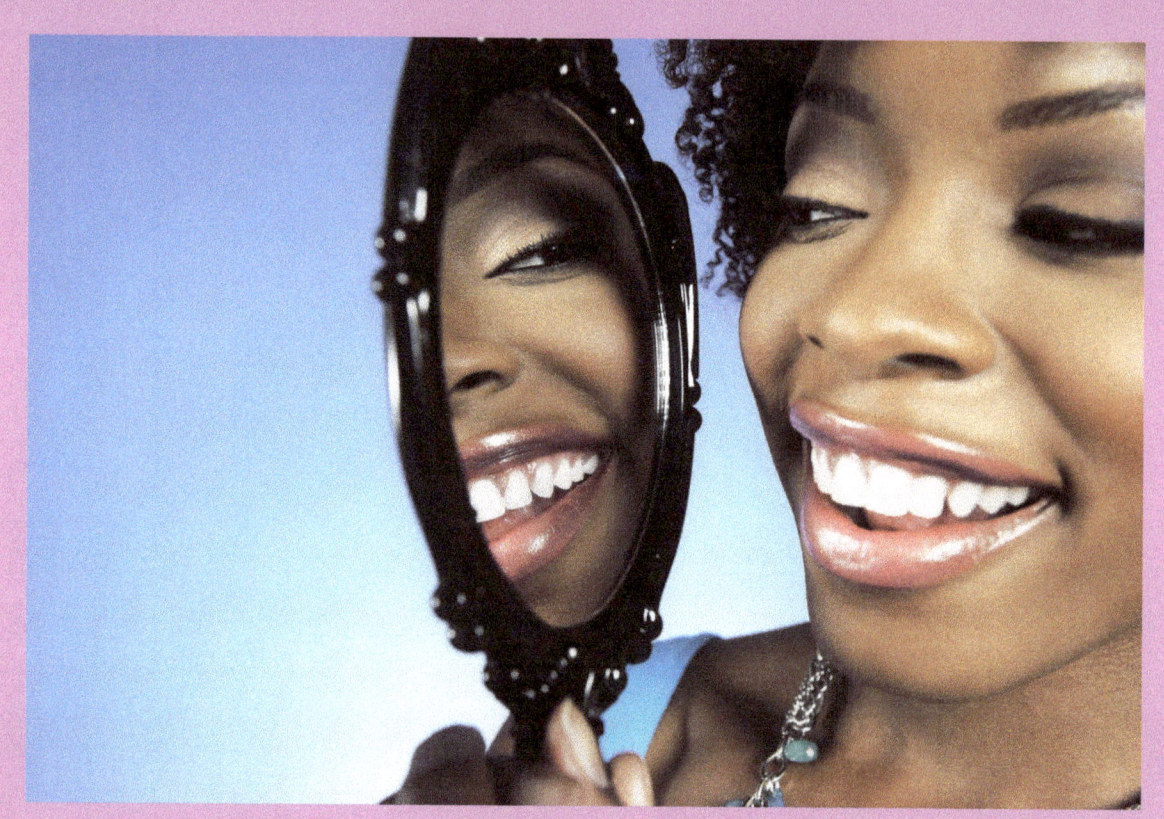

What do you see?

...Someone amazing smiling back at me.

Today I Also See...

Date:

___

Date:

___

Date:

___

Date:

___

WHEN I LOOK INTO THE MIRROR

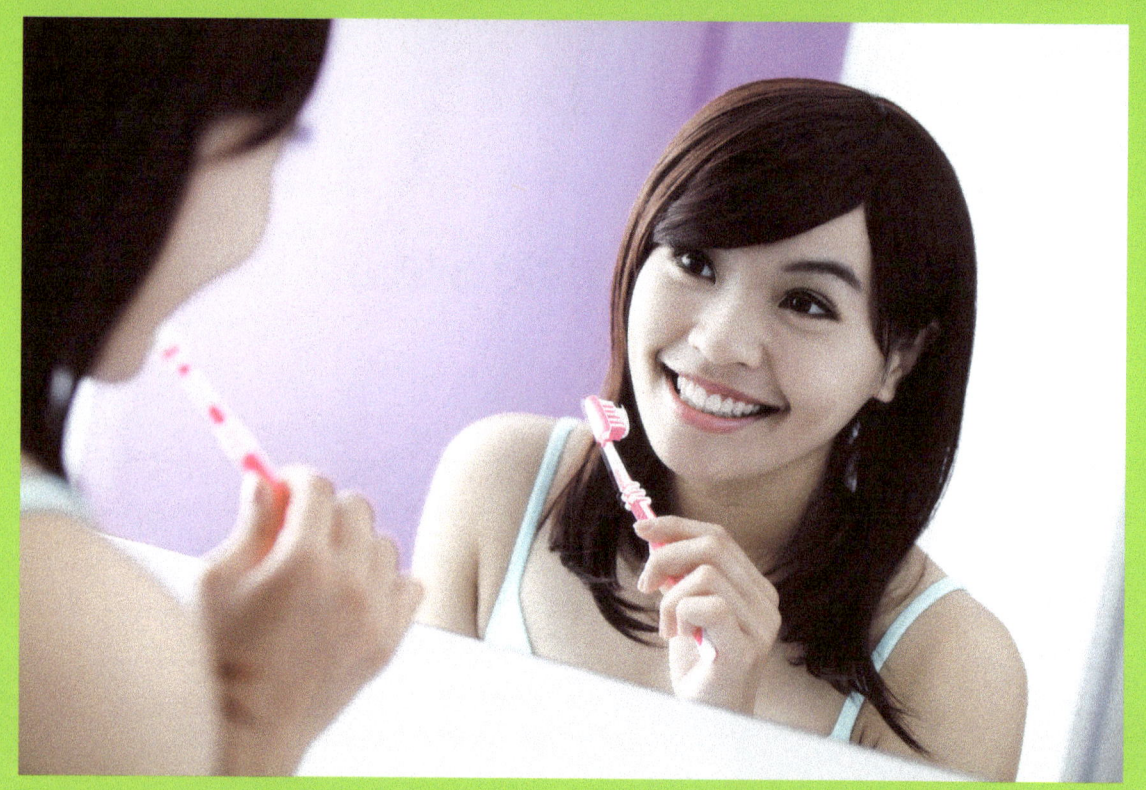

What do you see?

...Someone who has a positive influence over those around me.

Today I Also See...

Date:

___

Date:

___

Date:

___

Date:

___

WHEN I LOOK INTO THE MIRROR

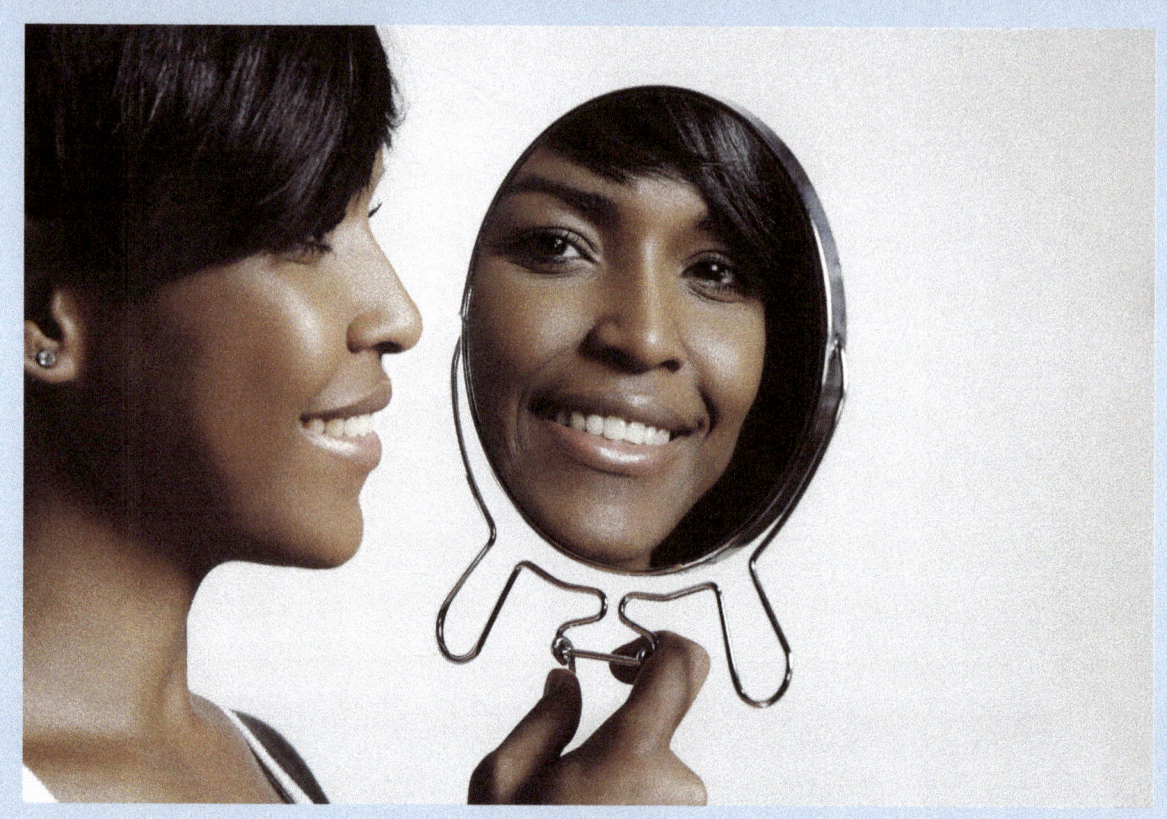

What do you see?

...I see a powerful person who is carefree.

Today I Also See...

Date:

___

Date:

___

Date:

___

Date:

___

WHEN I LOOK INTO THE MIRROR

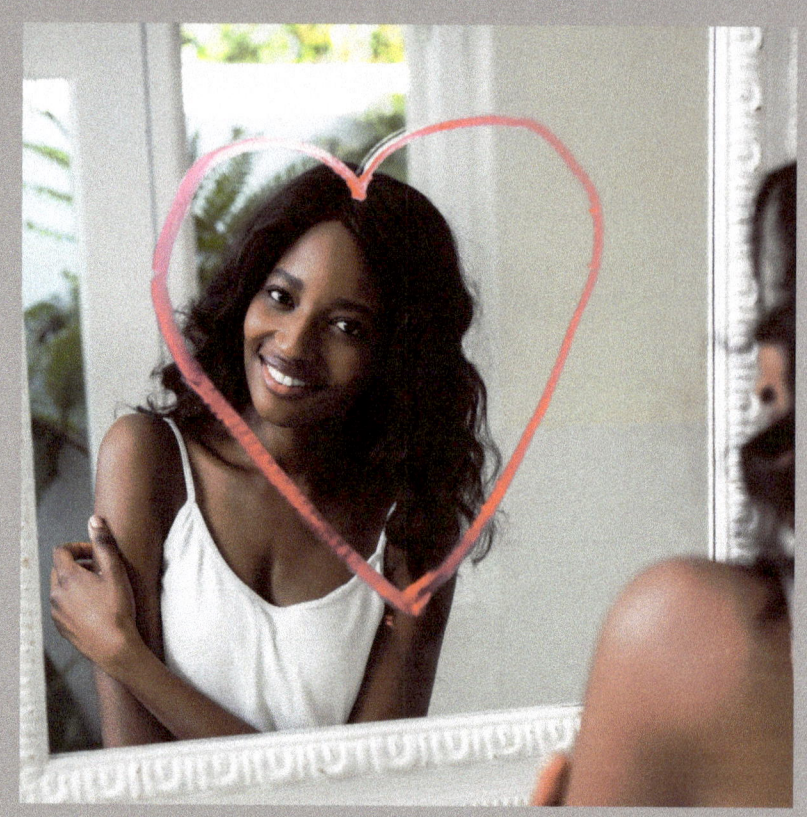

What do you see?

...A person who's always smiling and confirming oneself— who me.

Today I Also See...

Date:

Date:

Date:

Date:

WHEN I LOOK INTO THE MIRROR

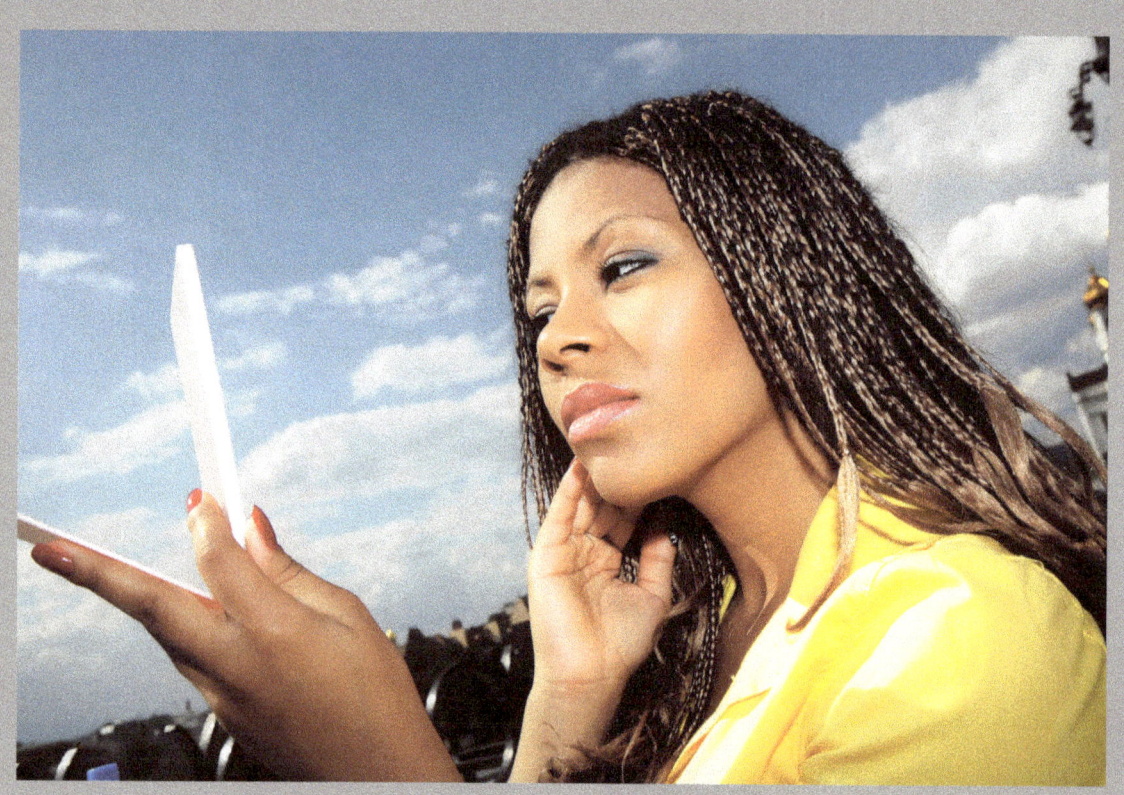

What do you see?

...My thoughts and dreams that are big enough to take me on the journey that God has planned just for me.

Today I Also See...

Date:

_____
_____
_____
_____
_____

Date:

_____
_____
_____
_____
_____

Date:

_____
_____
_____
_____
_____

Date:

_____
_____
_____
_____
_____

WHEN I LOOK INTO THE MIRROR

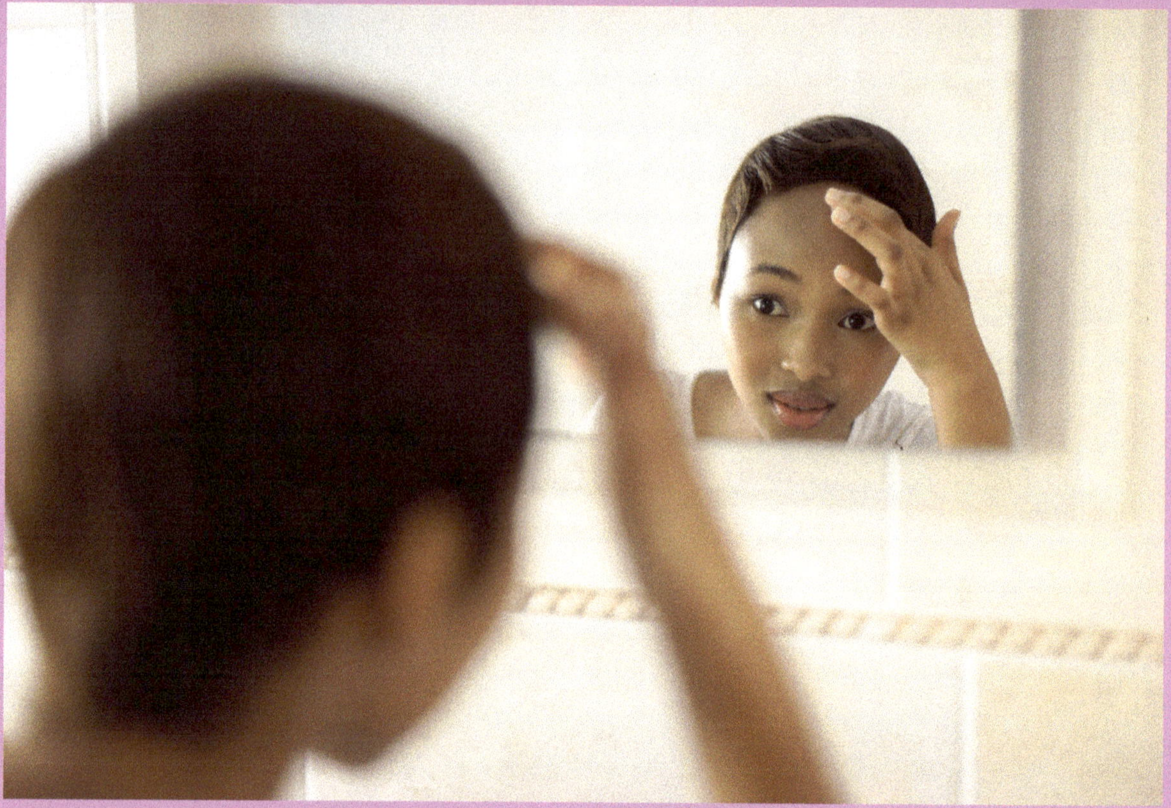

What do you see?

...My beautiful brown hair and eyes shining while others are admiring me.

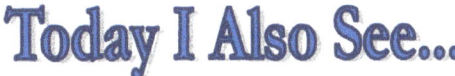
Today I Also See...

Date:
_____
_____
_____
_____
_____

Date:
_____
_____
_____
_____
_____

Date:
_____
_____
_____
_____
_____

Date:
_____
_____
_____
_____
_____

WHEN I LOOK INTO THE MIRROR

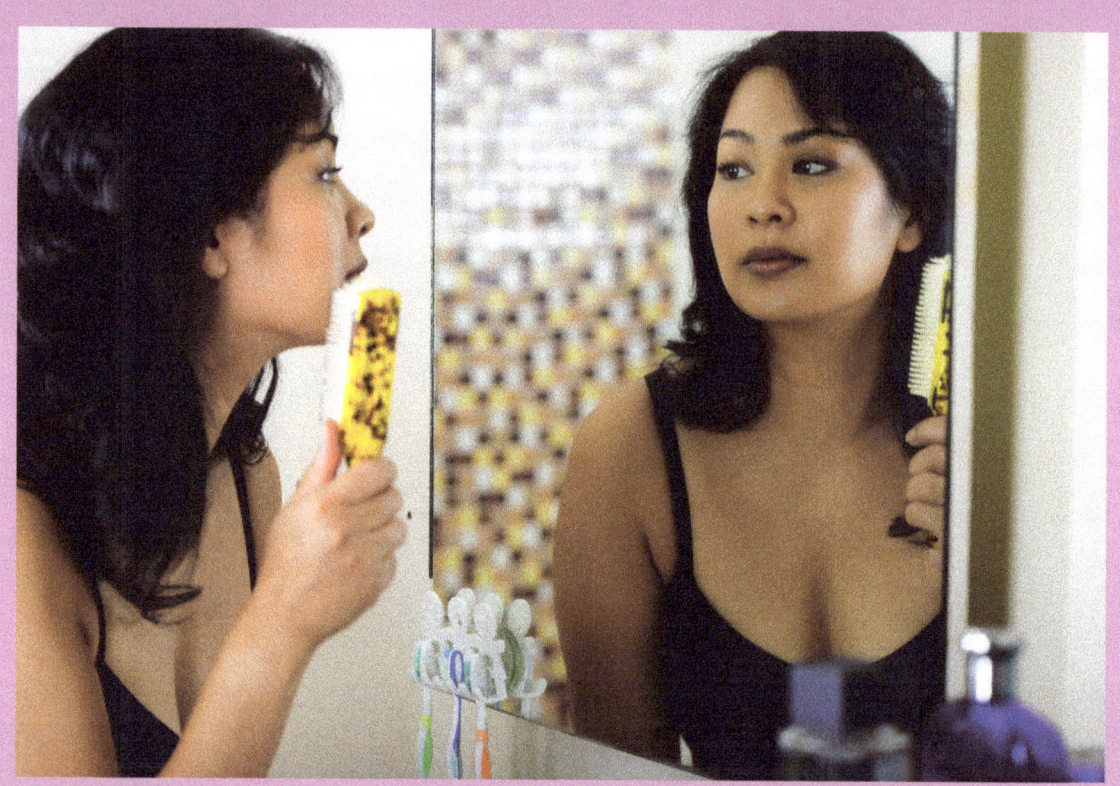

What do you see?

...Someone who's a little uncertain, yet excited about the future in front of me.

Today I Also See...

Date:

_____
_____
_____
_____
_____
_____

Date:

_____
_____
_____
_____
_____
_____

Date:

_____
_____
_____
_____
_____
_____

Date:

_____
_____
_____
_____
_____
_____

WHEN I LOOK INTO THE MIRROR

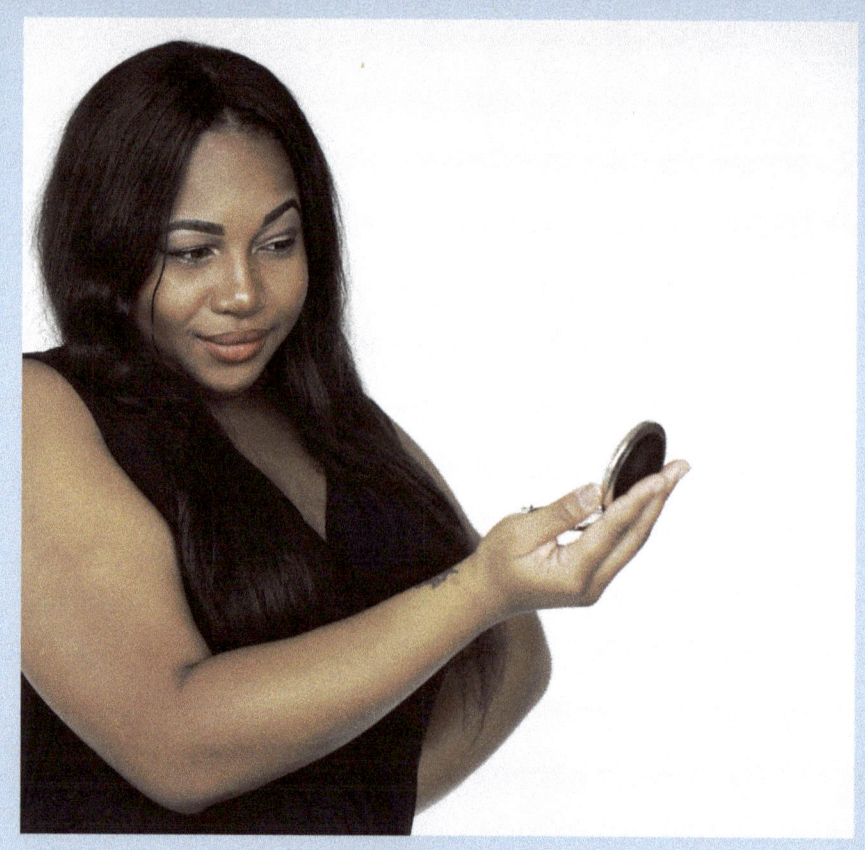

What do you see?

...Complete self-assurance and confidence all around me.

Today I Also See...

Date:

_____
_____
_____
_____
_____

Date:

_____
_____
_____
_____
_____

Date:

_____
_____
_____
_____
_____

Date:

_____
_____
_____
_____
_____

WHEN I LOOK INTO THE MIRROR

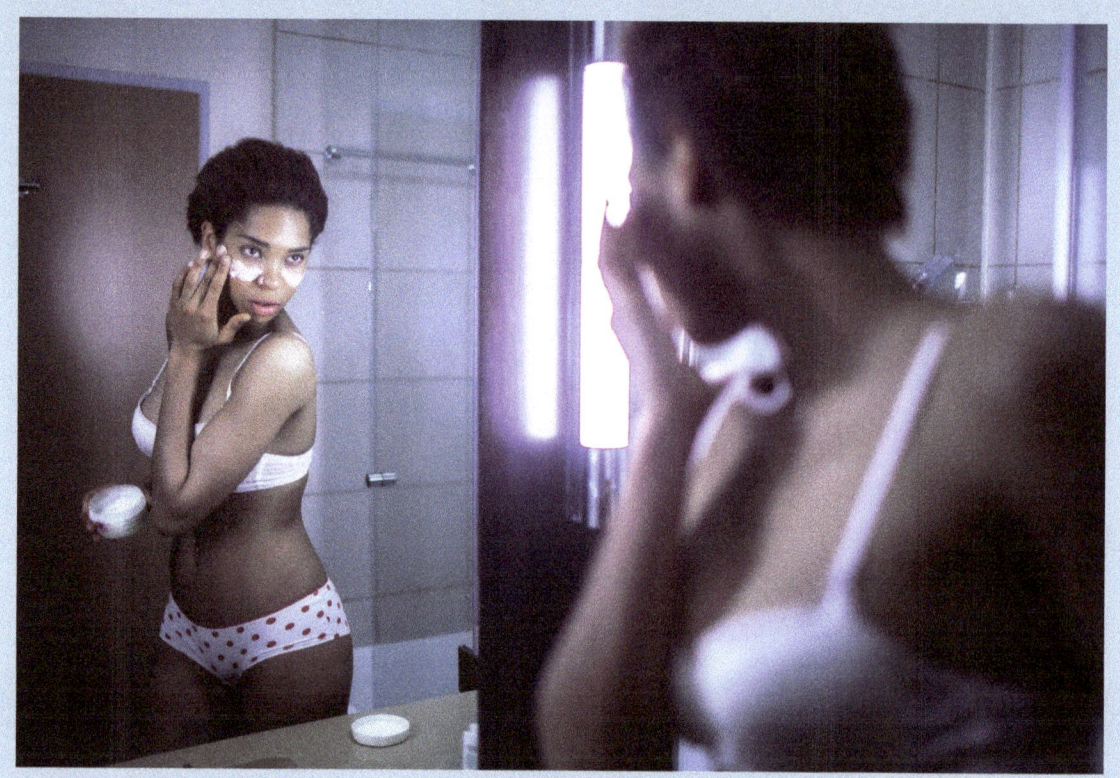

What do you see?

...A reflection of beauty: yes, it's me.

Today I Also See...

Date:

Date:

Date:

Date:

WHEN I LOOK INTO THE MIRROR

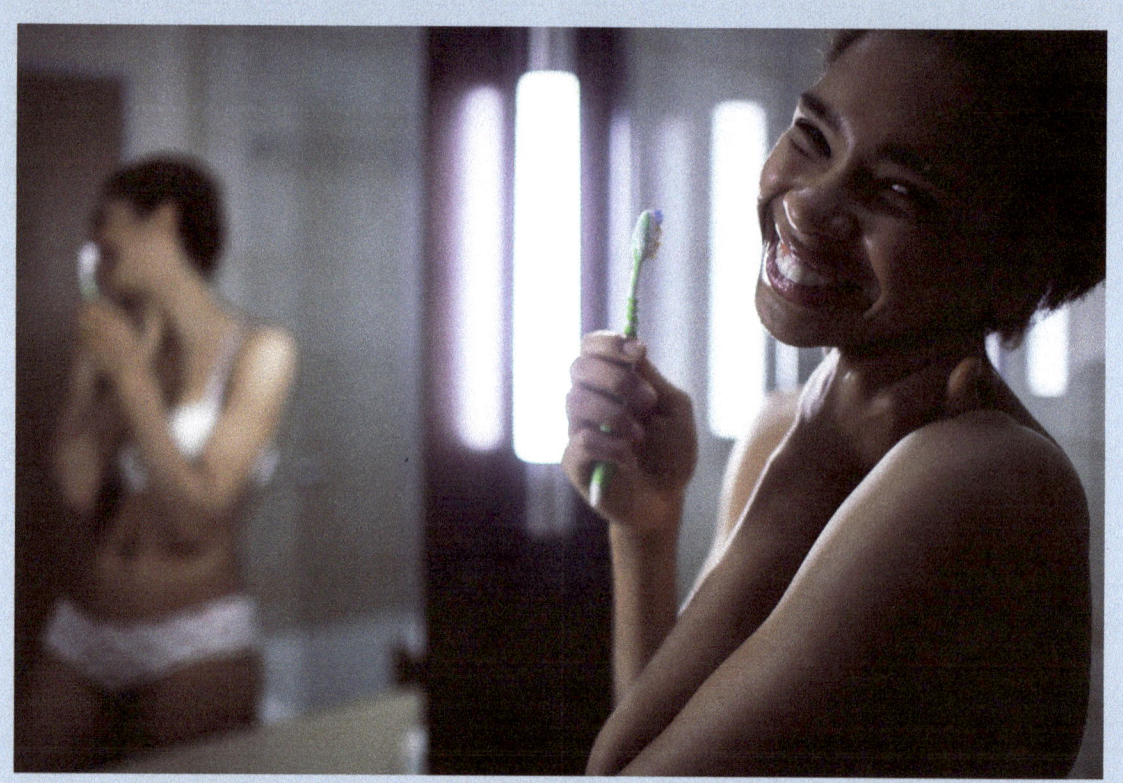

What do you see?

...Someone who is beginning to thrive,
WOW it's great to be me.

Today I Also See...

Date:

Date:

Date:

Date:

WHEN I LOOK INTO THE MIRROR

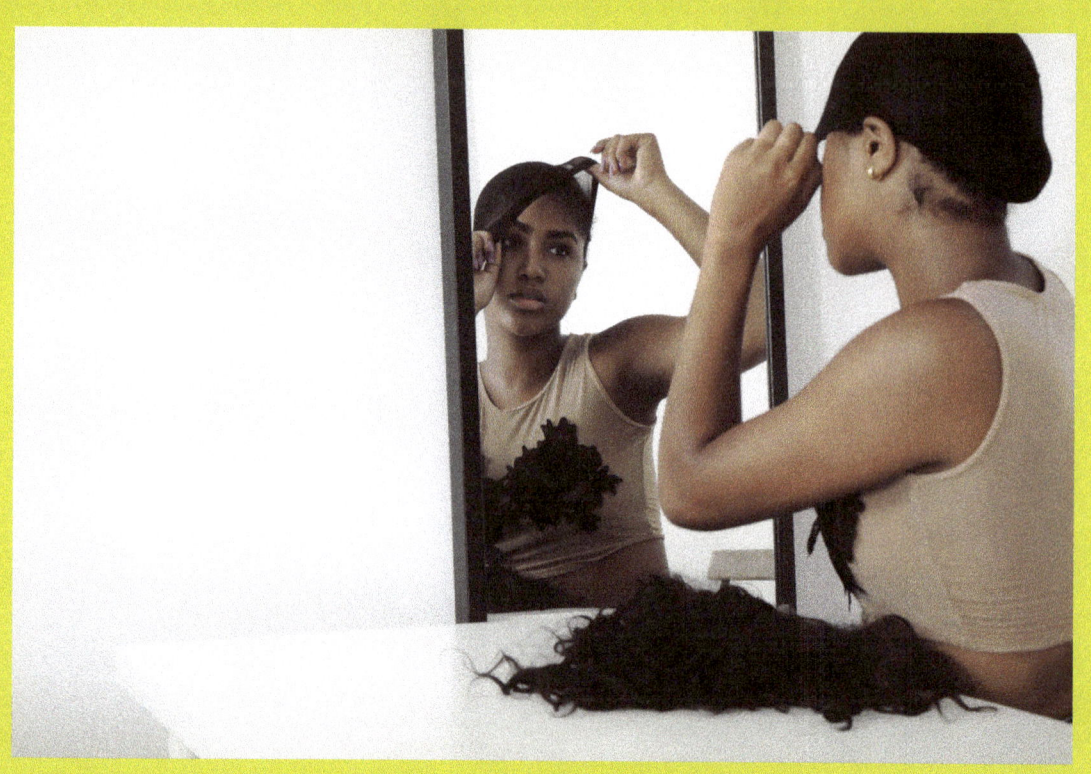

What do you see?

...Someone who is versatile
with total flexibility.

Today I Also See...

Date:
___
___
___
___
___

Date:
___
___
___
___
___

Date:
___
___
___
___
___

Date:
___
___
___
___
___

WHEN I LOOK INTO THE MIRROR

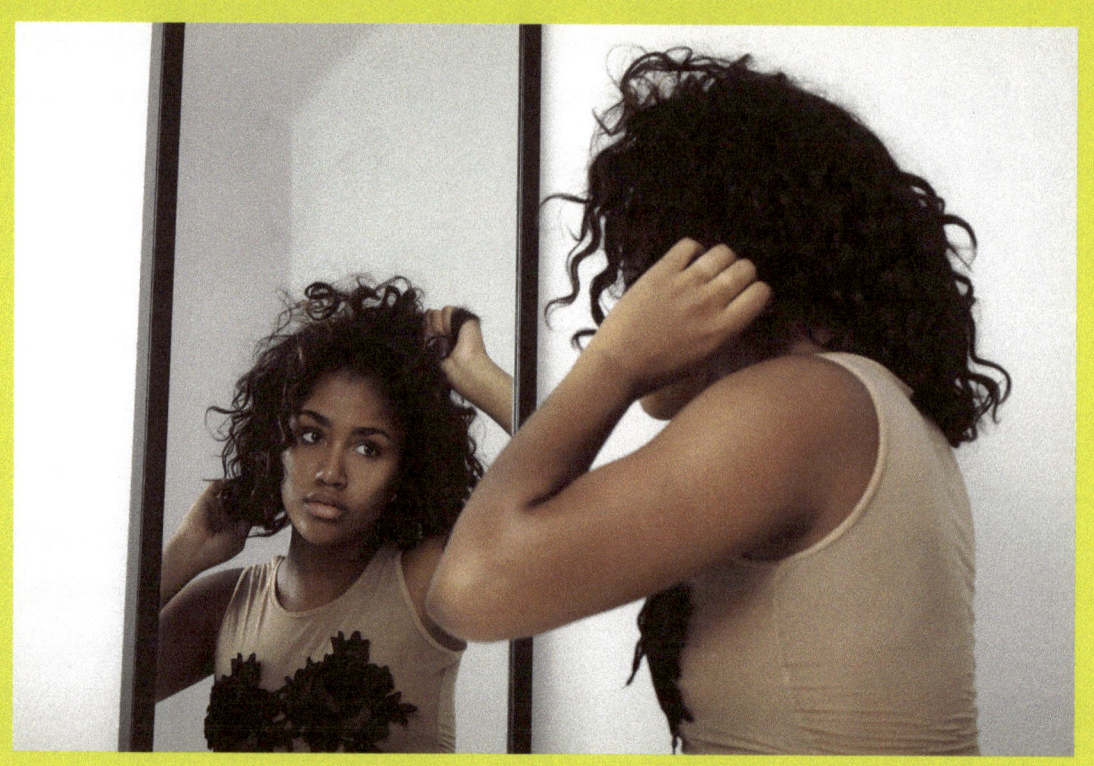

What do you see?

...That I am the only person who gets to choose how I define me.

Today I Also See...

Date:

_____
_____
_____
_____
_____
_____

Date:

_____
_____
_____
_____
_____
_____

Date:

_____
_____
_____
_____
_____
_____

Date:

_____
_____
_____
_____
_____
_____

WHEN I LOOK INTO THE MIRROR

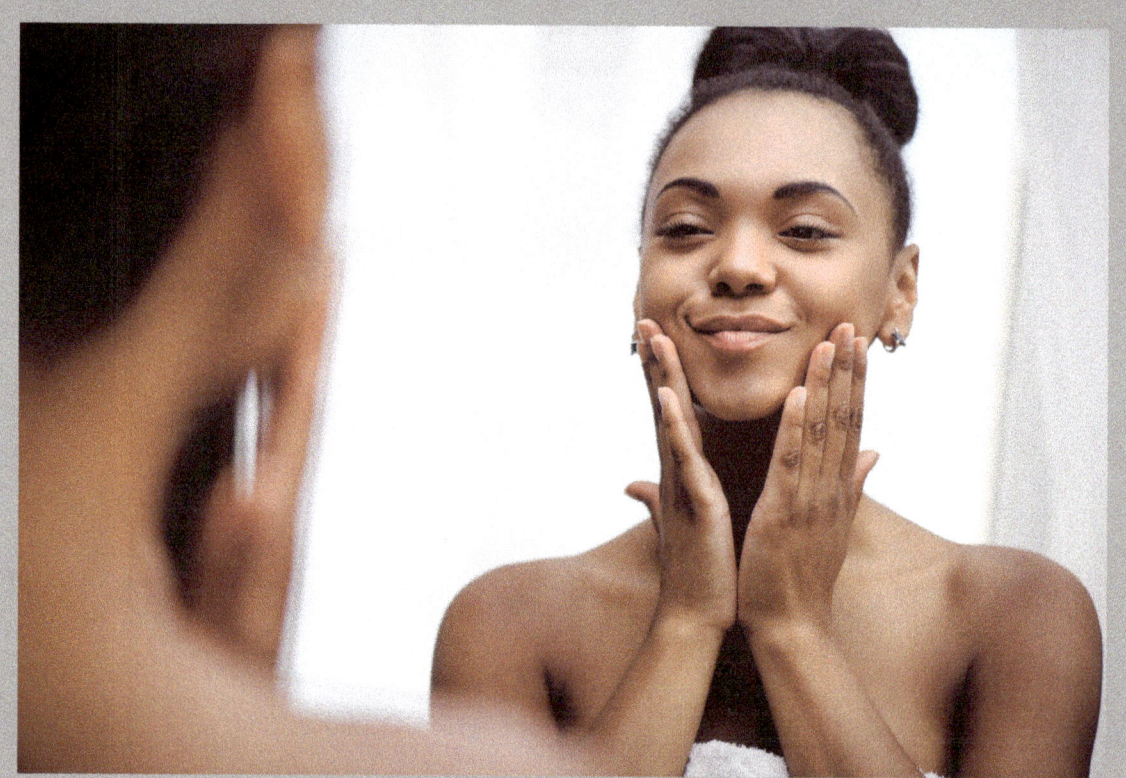

What do you see?

...The spirit of strong women of my family (ancestors) looking back at me.

Today I Also See...

Date:

_____
_____
_____
_____
_____

Date:

_____
_____
_____
_____
_____

Date:

_____
_____
_____
_____
_____

Date:

_____
_____
_____
_____
_____

WHEN I LOOK INTO THE MIRROR

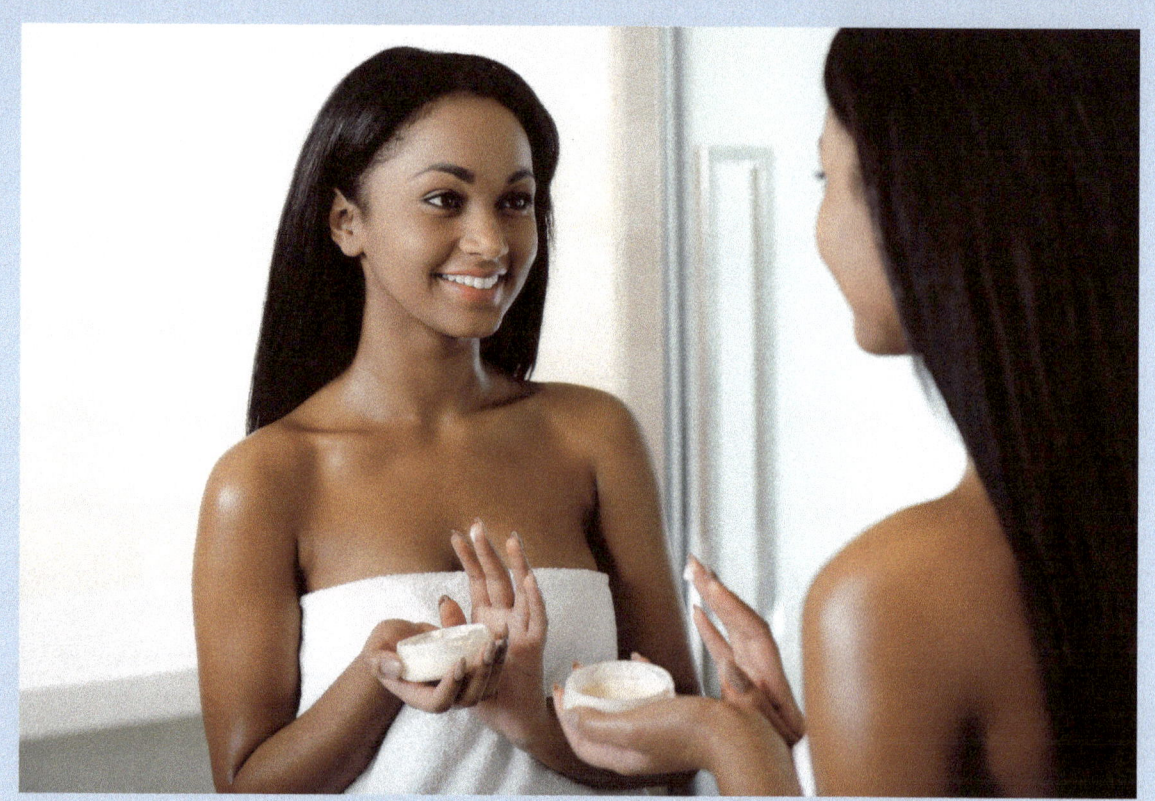

What do you see?

...The inner-beauty that is flawless that others too can see.

Today I Also See...

Date:

_____
_____
_____
_____
_____

Date:

_____
_____
_____
_____
_____

Date:

_____
_____
_____
_____
_____

Date:

_____
_____
_____
_____
_____

WHEN I LOOK INTO THE MIRROR

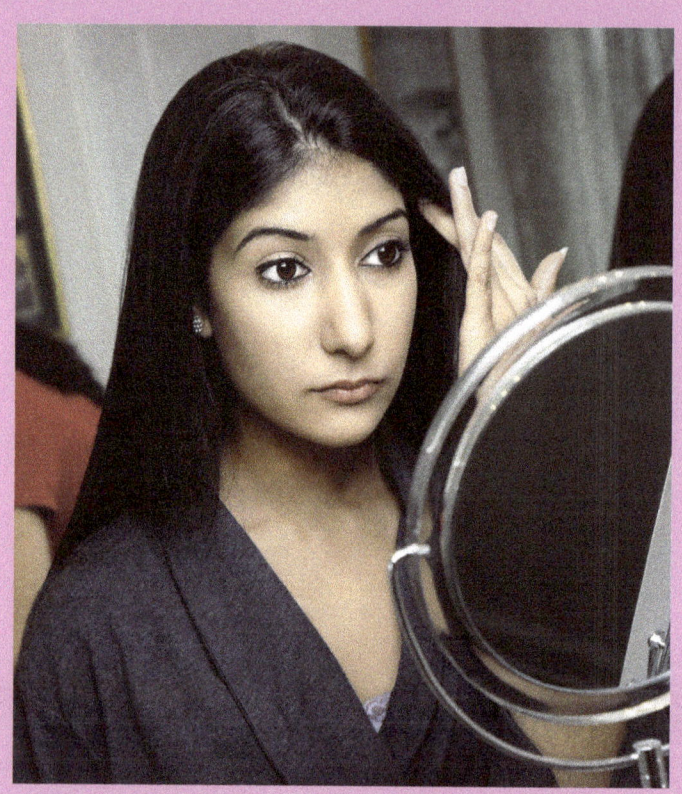

What do you see?

…The absolute goodness and joy of my Creator in me.

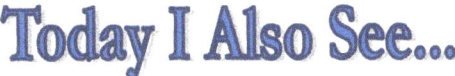

Today I Also See...

Date:

_____
_____
_____
_____
_____

Date:

_____
_____
_____
_____
_____

Date:

_____
_____
_____
_____
_____

Date:

_____
_____
_____
_____
_____

WHEN I LOOK INTO THE MIRROR

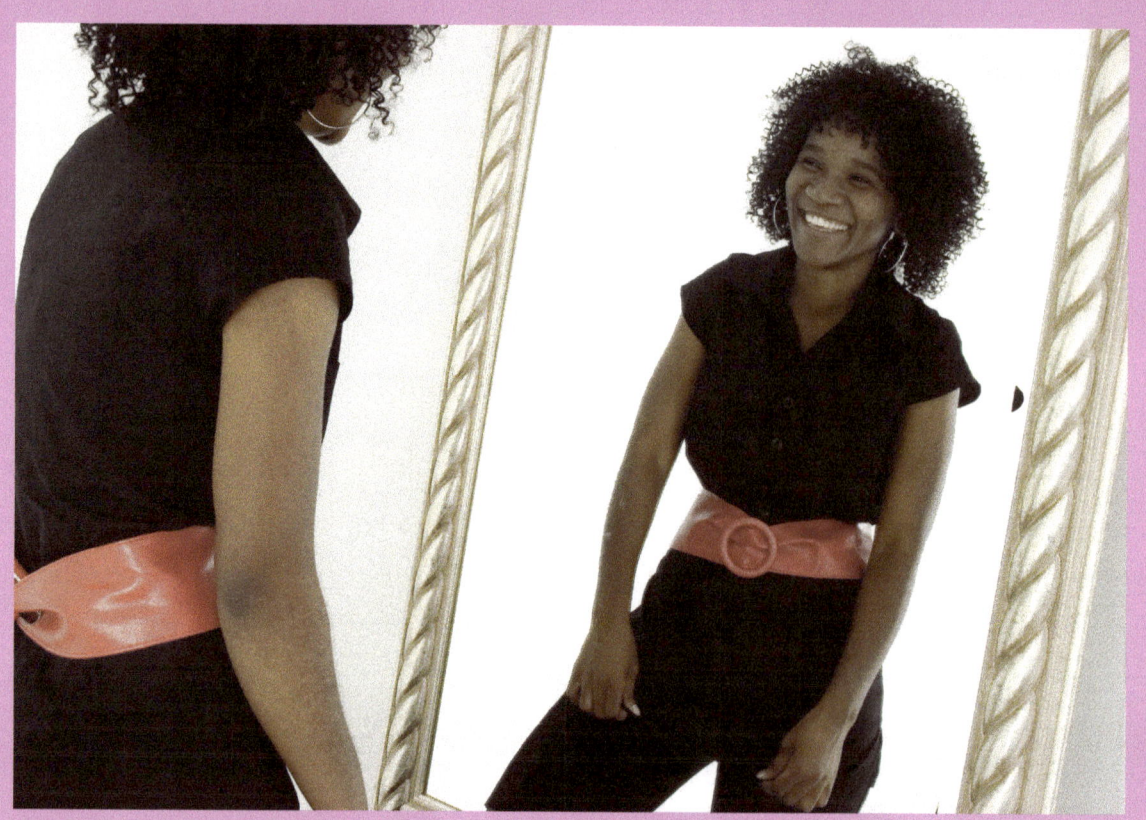

What do you see?

...Someone who is happy and go lucky!

Today I Also See...

Date:

_____
_____
_____
_____
_____
_____

Date:

_____
_____
_____
_____
_____
_____

Date:

_____
_____
_____
_____
_____
_____

Date:

_____
_____
_____
_____
_____
_____

WHEN I LOOK INTO THE MIRROR

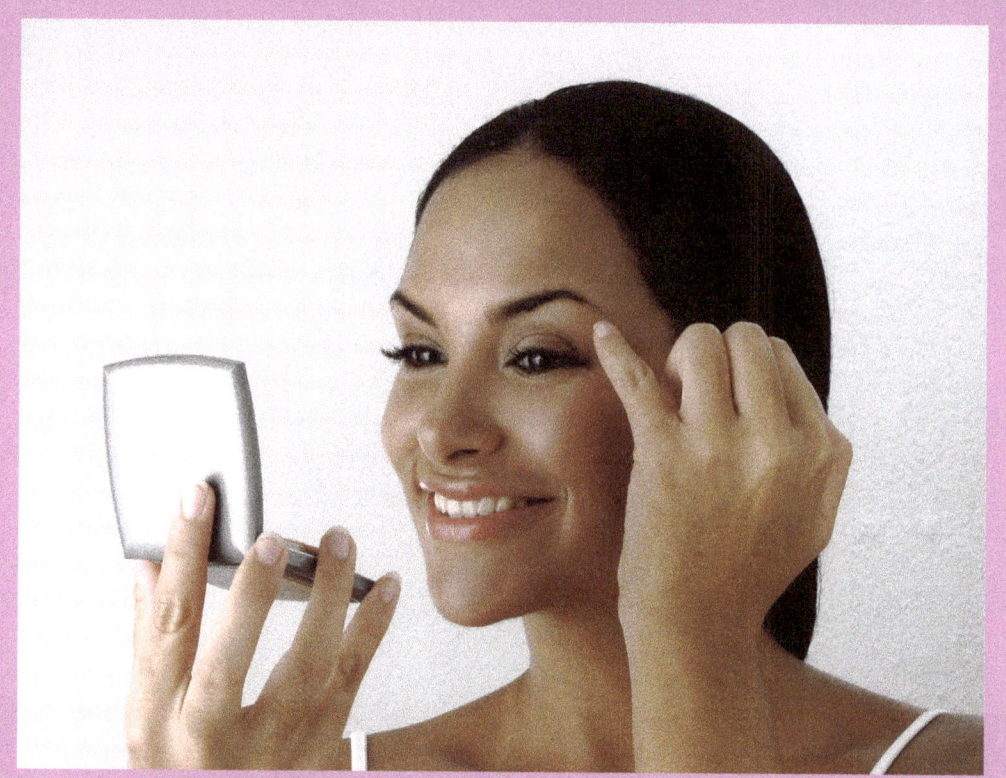

What do you see?

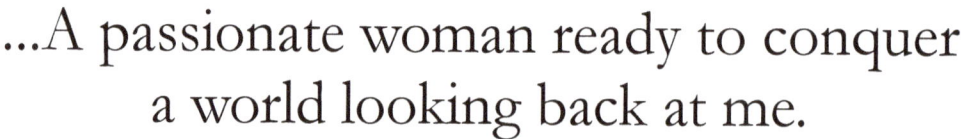

...A passionate woman ready to conquer
a world looking back at me.

Today I Also See...

Date:
_____
_____
_____
_____
_____
_____

Date:
_____
_____
_____
_____
_____
_____

Date:
_____
_____
_____
_____
_____
_____

Date:
_____
_____
_____
_____
_____
_____

WHEN I LOOK INTO THE MIRROR

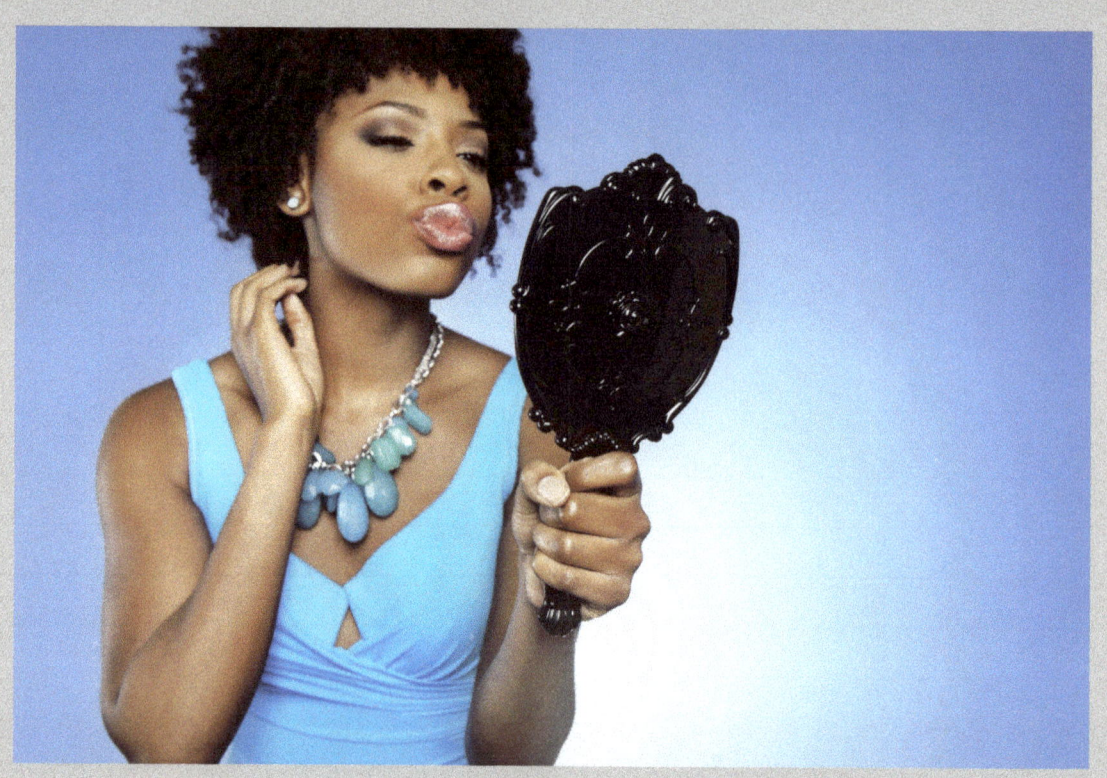

What do you see?

...Someone who is absolutely secure within me.

Today I Also See...

Date:

___

Date:

___

Date:

___

Date:

___

WHEN I LOOK INTO THE MIRROR

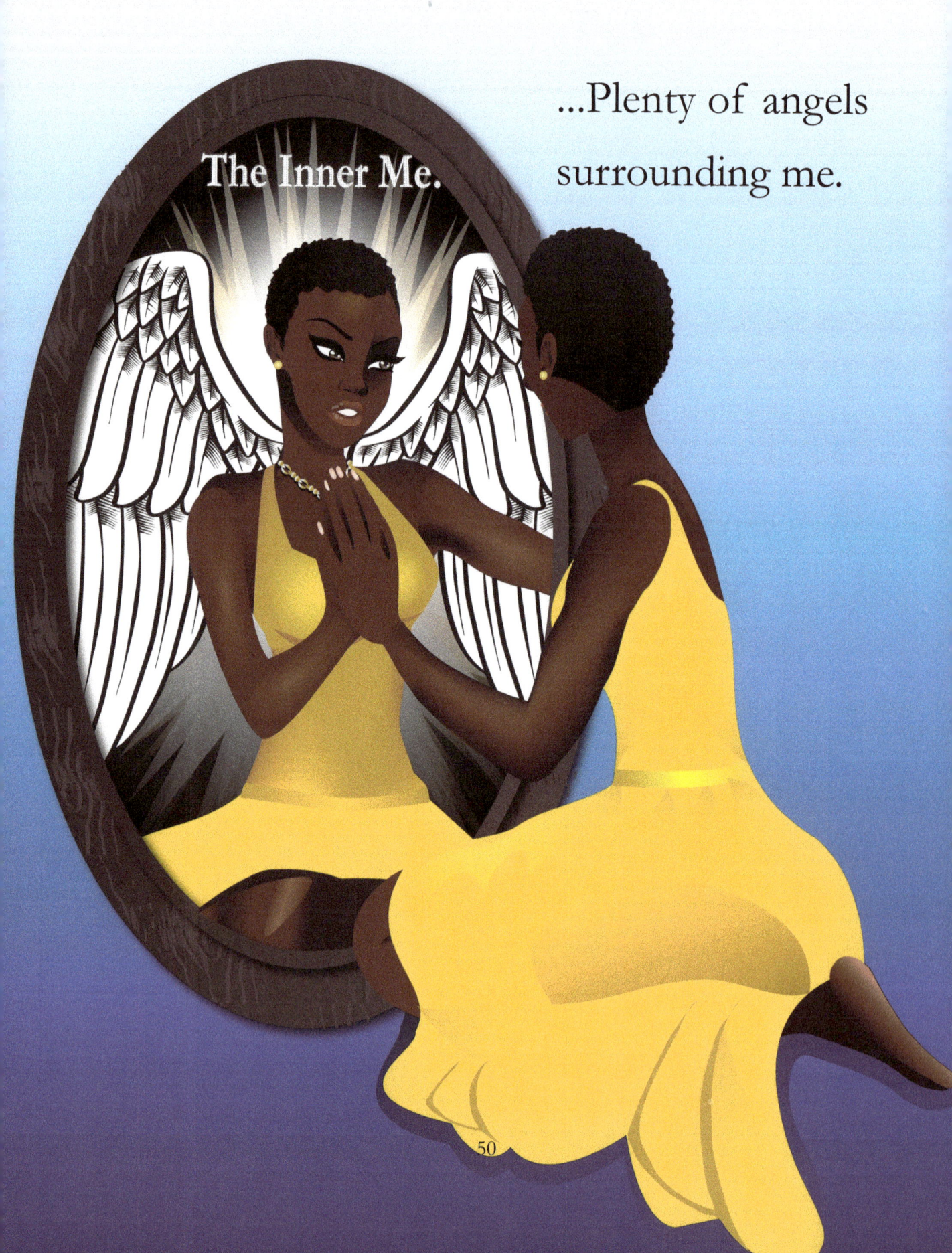

Today I Also See...

Date:

___

Date:

___

Date:

___

Date:

___

WHEN I LOOK INTO THE MIRROR

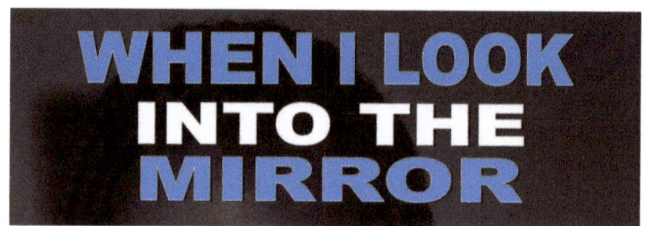

ABOUT THE AUTHOR

LaVon Jackson Maccanico lives in Arizona.

She is a wife, mother and grandmother who taught all of her children that they are healthy, beautiful, strong and smart. She constantly reminds them that they can do anything through Christ Jesus who strengthens them. She encourages them to find their inner strength and to be a positive influence in the lives of those who surround them.

One of her literary goals is to inspire all women of color and to let them know that they are healthy, beautiful, strong and smart, too.

www.ingramcontent.com/pod-product-compliance
Lightning Source LLC
LaVergne TN
LVHW070949070426
835507LV00029B/3460